Wall Pilates for Women:

A Transformative Challenge for Total Body Rejuvenation with Easy-to-Follow Illustrated Exercises for Beginners and All Skill Levels

Sawyer Foster

Table of Contents

Introduction

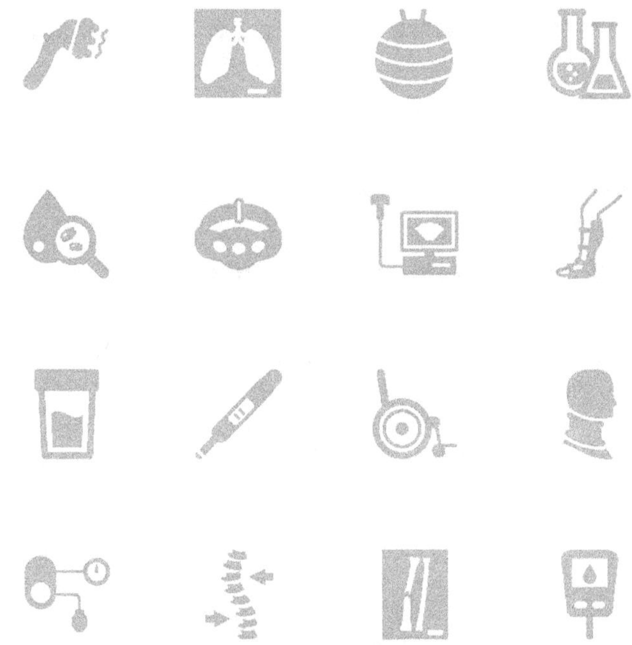

When we live in a world that is dominated by the rush and bustle of modern life, when stress is lurking around every corner and the demands on our time seem to never stop, it is easy to find ourselves feeling overwhelmed, physically depleted, and mentally exhausted. Take a moment to imagine a day that starts with a hurried breakfast, a race against the clock to meet deadlines, and a waterfall of duties that leaves you feeling as though you are juggling a thousand things at the same time. Don't you think it's a familiar sound? Every single one of us has experienced that.

Because of the commotion that is our everyday life, we frequently fail to pay attention to the basic foundation of our health, which is our bodies. It is the aches and pains that have become an unpleasant companion for many people that are the result of the toll that sedentary lives take, in conjunction with the tension that comes from having an endless list of things to do. However, what if I told you that there is a way that not only tackles the physical strains but also nurtures your emotional well-being? This is a holistic approach to fitness that has the potential to completely revolutionize your exercise routine. We are pleased to welcome you to the world of Wand Pilates, a journey that offers not just physical activity but also a change in living.

When you read these lines, think about the strain that builds up in your shoulders after a long day, the stiffness in your back that reminds you of the hours you spent sitting at your desk, or the mental exhaustion that makes it difficult for you to think clearly. Each and every one of us has been through this, and it is time that we acknowledge them. A sympathetic response to the silent cries of your body, Wand Pilates is a solution for the maladies that frequently go undiagnosed until they demand attention. Wand Pilates is not just another exercise routine; it is a compassionate answer to the silent cries of your body.

This is not a book about fast solutions or alleviation that is only used temporarily. Having a knowledge of your body, attending to its requirements, and cultivating a connection that is long-lasting between your physical and mental well-being are all important aspects. In order to embark on this adventure, you do not need to be a fitness guru or an experienced yogi. Wand Pilates is designed for everyone, regardless of age or fitness level, and will help you achieve your fitness goals. A guide to rediscovering the strength that is within you, both physically and mentally, in a manner that is easily incorporated into your daily routine, this book is a valuable resource.

As you continue to read through the pages that are to come, you will gradually become aware of the significant advantages that Wand Pilates may bring to your life. Imagining being able to say goodbye to the continuous back pain that is preventing you from being productive or experiencing an exciting surge of energy that helps you get through the day is a dream come true. Imagine a mind that is not clouded by stress but is clear, focused, and resilient in the face of obstacles. This is the mentality you should strive to manifest. Exactly this is the promise that Wand Pilates makes, a promise that is supported by an abundance of expertise and a profound comprehension of the challenges that you are facing.

With their extensive knowledge and experience in the field of holistic wellness, the author gives a fresh and original viewpoint to the field of fitness. It is sufficient to say that this person has devoted their entire life to the study and practice of mind-body connection, even though they have chosen not to reveal their identity. The author has seen the transformative impact of Wand Pilates in innumerable lives, including their own, and thanks to their years of experience, they have observed this power firsthand. The knowledge that is shared in this book is not only theoretical; rather, it is the conclusion of practical insights. These insights were obtained through years of diligent investigation and a true enthusiasm for assisting others in achieving success.

Pilates with a Wand is not a solution that is universally applicable. Rather than that, it provides a personalized approach, acknowledging that every body is different and calls for individualized care. By reading this book, you will get a profound comprehension of the fundamental ideas that underpin Wand Pilates, as well as the ability to modify those principles to meet your own requirements. There will be no more generic workout regimens that leave you feeling disconnected; this is a voyage of self-discovery that connects with the rhythm of your body and promotes a sense of harmony via the process of working out.

If you have ever had a need for a change, for a more comprehensive approach to physical training that goes beyond the superficial, then Wand Pilates is the solution you have been looking for. This is not merely a book; rather, it is a guide, a partner on your quest to rediscover the power, flexibility, and resilience that are already there within you. As you progress through the book, you will come to the realization that this is not only a workout regimen; rather, it is a transformative experience that goes beyond the physical and touches the very essence of your being. You are about to start on a journey of self-discovery, where the magic of Wand Pilates will emerge, providing you with a road to a life that is healthier, happier, and more balanced that you have never experienced before.

Chapter 1:

History and origins of Wand Pilates

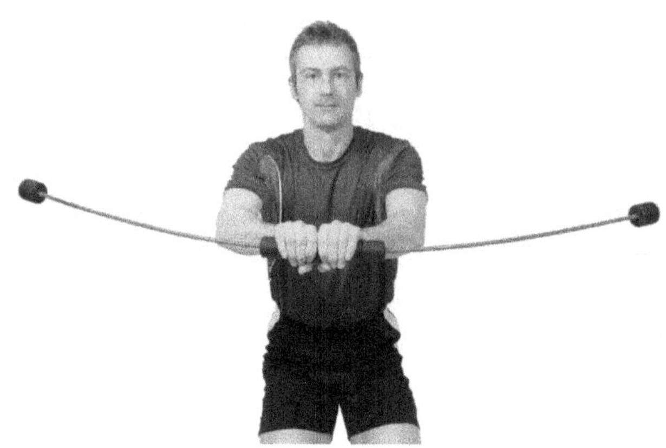

Since it was first introduced in the early 20th century, Pilates, which is a holistic approach to physical health, has seen continuous development. The technique, which was first referred to as "Contrology," was initially established by Joseph Pilates. Its primary objective was to foster the integration of the mind and body through a series of regulated movements. Pilates's success in developing core strength, flexibility, and overall body awareness has contributed to the widespread adoption of this exercise technique over the years.

As the Pilates method has continued to develop, numerous modifications and pieces of apparatus have been developed in order to broaden the range of exercises and increase their intensity. An example of such a change is the addition of a wand, which is a piece of equipment that provides Pilates routines with an additional dimension. In order to acquire an understanding of the advantages and distinctive characteristics of Wand Pilates, it is necessary to investigate the history and origins of Pilates in general.

While serving in the military during World War I, Joseph Pilates, a fitness enthusiast from Germany, devised the Pilates method as a means of rehabilitating injured soldiers. Pilates, which was modelled after other forms of exercise such as yoga, gymnastics, and martial arts, was developed with the intention of developing a comprehensive system that addressed both physical and mental well-being. Over the course of the 1920s, Pilates founded his first studio in New York City, where his method achieved widespread popularity.

The Pilates practice has remained centered on the fundamental concepts that underpin it, which include concentration, control, centering, precision, breath, and flow. On the other hand, as Pilates gained popularity, practitioners and teachers started experimenting with diverse versions to accommodate a wide range of fitness levels and personal preferences.

In the past few decades, the fitness industry has witnessed a significant increase in the utilization of various props and pieces of apparatus in the context of classic Pilates workouts. These augmentations are designed to offer supplementary resistance, support, or help, with the ultimate goal of boosting the overall effectiveness of the exercises. The wand, which is sometimes referred to as a Pilates stick or magic circle, is one of these pieces of equipment that has become increasingly popular within the Pilates community.

The wand that is utilized in Pilates is often made out of a rod made of metal or fiberglass that is lightweight and flexible. For the purpose of comfort, the rod is frequently wrapped in foam or rubber. The length of the wand can vary, and according to the manufacturer, it may come with resistance settings that can be adjusted to match a variety of fitness levels. A new dynamic is introduced into Pilates with the addition of the wand, which challenges the body in ways that are not found in other forms of exercise and targets specific muscle groups.

Benefits of Incorporating a Wand into Pilates

The incorporation of a wand into Pilates routines results in a plethora of benefits. These benefits include the combination of the fundamentals of Pilates with the additional resistance and versatility of the prop. A number of the most important benefits are:

1. Pilates, in its traditional form, already has an emphasis on core activation, but this is enhanced by the Pilates method. The addition of the wand results in an additional layer of resistance, which necessitates higher steadiness and control. In order to do this, the core muscles, which include the abdominals, obliques, and lower back, are engaged in a more intensive manner during the exercises that are performed with the wand.

2. Increased Flexibility: The wand makes it possible to perform specific exercises with a greater range of motion, which results in increased flexibility. The controlled movements that are done with the wand facilitate the elongation of muscles, which, with time, contributes to improvements in flexibility and joint mobility.

3. Improved Posture: A significant number of Pilates exercises concentrate on correct alignment and posture, and the wand acts as a tactile signal to improve one's awareness of their body. It is possible for practitioners to obtain improved spine alignment, shoulder placement, and general posture by using the wand as a guide.

4. Targeted Muscle Engagement: The wand makes it possible to precisely target particular muscle groups that need to be worked. It doesn't matter if you're working out your arms, legs, or back; the resistance that the wand offers makes it

possible to engage your muscles in a concentrated manner, which in turn makes your workout more efficient and effective.

5. Wand Pilates allows for a broad variety of different exercises to be performed, which brings about a great deal of versatility. The prop adds diversity to workouts, which helps practitioners stay interested and motivated. This can be accomplished by incorporating the wand into standard Pilates mat exercises or by designing whole new motions.

6. Through the provision of resistance in both pushing and pulling motions, the wand can be utilized to treat muscular imbalances, hence facilitating the development of balanced strength. With this well-rounded strategy, you may rest assured that opposing muscle groups will be trained proportionally, hence lowering the likelihood of injury.

7. The focused nature of Pilates is further enhanced when a wand is utilized, which is consistent with the mind-body connection. Within the Pilates technique, practitioners are required to concentrate on regulated movements, awareness of the breath, and exact muscle engagement in order to strengthen the mind-body connection that is intrinsic to the discipline.

Overview of the Unique Features of Wand Pilates

One of the ways that Wand Pilates differentiates itself from regular Pilates is by utilizing a prop that is both straightforward and efficient. Its popularity and effectiveness in increasing total fitness and well-being are largely attributable to the distinctive characteristics of Wand Pilates, which are as follows:

1. The shape of the wand makes it portable and easy to transport, which enables folks

to practice Pilates nearly anywhere. Additionally, the wand is lightweight. The fact that it is lightweight makes it possible for a wide variety of people, regardless of their age or level of physical fitness, to use it.

2. Adjustable Resistance: Many wands come equipped with resistance levels that can be adjusted, enabling users to tailor the level of difficulty of their exercises to their own needs. Because of this aspect, Wand Pilates is suited for a wide range of practitioners, including those who are just starting out as well as those who have more experience.

3. Application Flexibility: The wand can be incorporated into a wide variety of Pilates exercises, both on the mat and with other pieces of Pilates apparatus. Because of its adaptability, practitioners are able to target different muscle groups and tailor their routines to individual fitness goals.

4. Enhanced Stability and Support: In addition to providing more resistance, the wand can also be utilized as a tool for enhancing stability during specific workouts. The practitioners are able to receive more assistance when it is required, while at the same time successfully exercising their muscles thanks to this dual functioning.

5. Engagement of the Upper and Lower Bodies Wand Pilates is a form of exercise that involves both the upper and lower body, which allows for a more comprehensive engagement of the muscles. The utilization of this full-body method guarantees a comprehensive workout, which in turn encourages the development of balanced strength and coordination.

6. The usage of the wand necessitates a higher level of attention and mindfulness during the exercises. Mindful movement and concentration are also required. In order to reinforce the fundamental concepts of Pilates, practitioners are required

to place a strong emphasis on retaining control, maintaining perfect form, and moving in a deliberate manner.

7. Creative Exercise Variations: When it comes to Wand Pilates, instructors and practitioners have the ability to put their creative skills to use by coming up with novel exercises and sequences to keep workouts exciting and challenging. This adaptability is among the factors that contribute to the continued development of Pilates as a dynamic and ever-evolving form of physical exercise.

Wand Pilates is a contemporary development of the conventional Pilates method. It is characterized by the incorporation of a versatile and efficient prop that serves to improve the overall experience of working out. There are a multitude of advantages that come with the utilization of the wand, including enhanced core activation, enhanced flexibility, and balanced strength development. Pilates is made available to a wider audience thanks to the wand's portable and customizable qualities, which also contribute to the development of a more conscious and holistic approach to physical training. Wand Pilates is a dynamic and engaging variant that contributes to the ongoing heritage of this transformative exercise system. As Pilates continues to evolve, Wand Pilates stands out as a variation that contributes to this legacy.

Chapter 2:

Choosing the Right Wand

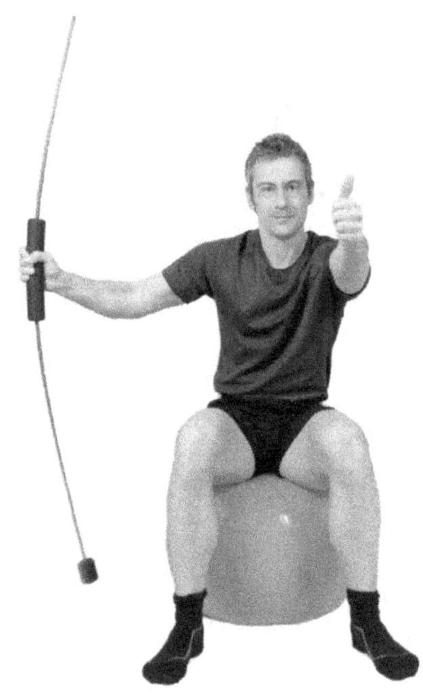

When it comes to the enchanted realm of magic, a wizard's wand is more than simply a tool; it is an extension of their magical abilities and a reflection of who they are as a person. In order to become a successful wizard or witch, one of the most important steps is to choose the appropriate wand. In this chapter, we will discuss the numerous types of wands that are available, the significance of selecting the wand that is suitable for one's specific requirements, as well as the factors that should be taken into consideration about the appropriate size and weight.

Types of Wands Available

Similar like the people who wield them, wands are available in a wide range of shapes, sizes, and materials. Every single wand is one of a kind, with its own set of magical qualities and qualities that are unique to it. These are some of the most prevalent kinds of wands.:

1. **Wood Types:**

   - *Wands made of oak, which is well-known for its strength and longevity, are frequently preferred by wizards who have a penchant for more traditional and stable wands.*

   - *Willow: Willow wands are exceptionally useful for spellwork that involves healing and charms because of their flexibility and resilience.*

   - *The type of wood known as hawthorn is frequently connected with intricate and potent magic, making it an ideal choice for more experienced spellcasters.*

2. **Core Materials:**

   - *Feather of the Phoenix: Wands that have phoenix feather cores are renowned for their impressive and adaptable magical properties. Those who have a natural flair for casting spells frequently choose them as their spellcasting companions.*

   - *Dragon Heartstring: Dragon heartstring cores offer a balance of power and control, which is why they are so popular among wizards who are looking for precision in their spellwork.*

   - *Wands that have cores made of unicorn hair are recognized for their devotion, and they are frequently preferred by individuals who place a high emphasis on having a strong connection with their specific magical instrument.*

3. **Length:**

   - Wands can range in length from short to lengthy, and the length that a wizard chooses to use is frequently determined by their personality and personal preferences. Wands that are shorter may allow greater control, while wands that are longer may bring about an increase in the magical reach..

4. **Flexibility:**

   - In addition to this, the adaptability of a wand is an essential component. While there are wands that are hard and provide focused and direct magic, there are also wands that are more flexible and allow for a wider variety of applications.

In order to select a wand that is in harmony with the magical tendencies and personality of the person who will be wielding it, it is vital to have a thorough understanding of the many combinations of wood kinds, core materials, length, and flexibility.

Selecting the Appropriate Wand for Individual Needs

Due to the fact that the relationship between a wizard and their wand is comparable to that of a magical symbiosis, selecting the appropriate wand is a complex and deeply personal procedure. When choosing the right wand for your specific requirements, it is important to bear the following things in mind:

1. **Magical Affinities:**

   - There are many different kinds of magic that wizards have a preference for learning. While some people may be particularly skilled in charms and enchantments, others may be more inclined to focus on defensive spells or elemental magic. A person's total spellcasting powers can be improved by selecting a wand that is complementary to their magical innate abilities.

2. **Personality Traits:**

   - It is stated that wands select their owners based on the characteristics of their personalities. In the same way that a more restrained person might connect with a wand that resonates with subtlety and refinement, a wizard who is daring and adventurous might find a wand that shares the qualities they are looking for.

3. **Magical Goals:**

   - Long-term magical objectives are something that should be taken into consideration by a wizard. In the event that a wizard had the goal of becoming an expert potion maker, it is possible that a wand that excels in precision and subtlety would be more ideal than one that is geared toward raw force.

4. **Compatibility:**

   - In order for a wizard to successfully cast spells, it is vital that the wizard and their wand are compatible with one another. As if the wand itself were an extension of the wizard's magical nature, wizards frequently experience a resonance or connection when they find the wand that best suits their needs.

5. **Trial and Error:**

   - It is not unusual for wizards to experiment with a number of different wands until they locate the one that is the most comfortable to use. It is possible that some wizards will experience a connection right away, while others may require some time to try with several wands in order to find the one that is most effectively suited to their needs.

In the end, the process of choosing the perfect wand is a journey of self-discovery for the wizard. It gives them the opportunity to investigate and comprehend their magical identity on a more profound level.

Proper Sizing and Weight Considerations

When it comes to a wizard's ability to efficiently handle a wand, the physical characteristics of the wand, like as its size and weight, have a vital importance. When it comes to spellcasting, these considerations are very necessary in order to achieve precision and control:

1. **Length:**

   - The range and power of the spells that a wand is capable of casting are directly influenced by the length of the wand. When it comes to spellwork, those who place a higher priority on precision and control tend to select shorter wands, while those who prefer longer wands look for those that provide enhanced reach and strength. It is important for wizards to select a length that is compatible with the casting manner that they favor.

2. **Weight:**

   - It is also important to consider the weight of a wand when determining whether or not a wizard will be able to comfortably hold it. A wand that is too heavy may cause weariness during extended spellcasting sessions, but a wand that is too light may not have the proper heft for some spells. Both of these aspects of the wand are important to consider. The goal of wizards should be to find a balance that is not only pleasant but also enables them to maintain their concentrate on magic.

3. **Grip:**

   - It is common practice to disregard the grip of a wand, despite the fact that it is vital for retaining control while performing spells. For optimal performance, wizards should select a wand that has a grip that is both comfortable and secure in their hands. There are wands that have intricate designs or textures on the handle, which adds a touch of individuality and customization to the product.

4. **Balance:**

- The degree to which a wand's weight is distributed is what determines its equilibrium. Having a wand that is well-balanced facilitates the passage of magic from the wizard through the wand in a manner that is uninterrupted and precise. It is important for wizards to try out a variety of wands in order to locate the one that best suits their magical style so that they can use it.

5. **Versatility:**

- The adaptability of the wand is something that have to be taken into consideration. While there are wands that are designed to be used for particular kinds of magic, there are also wands that are more versatile and can be used for a wide range of spells. One type of wand may be chosen by a wizard to serve as their primary focus, while another type of wand may be chosen to serve as a backup for a variety of magical requirements.

It is vital for a wizard to take into consideration the appropriate dimensions and weight of their wand in order to use it with skill and expertise. With the right combination of elements, a wand can become an extension of the wizard, enabling them to channel their magical energy with greater precision and dexterity.

An important turning point in the life of a witch or wizard is when they select the appropriate wand. This event signifies the beginning of a magical journey, a collaboration between the spellcaster and the instrument that they have chosen to represent them.

Acquiring an understanding of the many sorts of wands, picking the wand that is most suitable for one's specific requirements, and taking into consideration the optimum sizing and weight are all essential components of this procedure.

During the course of their search for the ideal wand, wizards not only come across a potent magical instrument, but they also come across a reflection of their own identity and the potential they possess. A companion that assists the wizard in their quest for magical knowledge and mastery, the wand becomes an integral part of the wizard's life.

Chapter 3:

Fundamental Wand Pilates Exercises

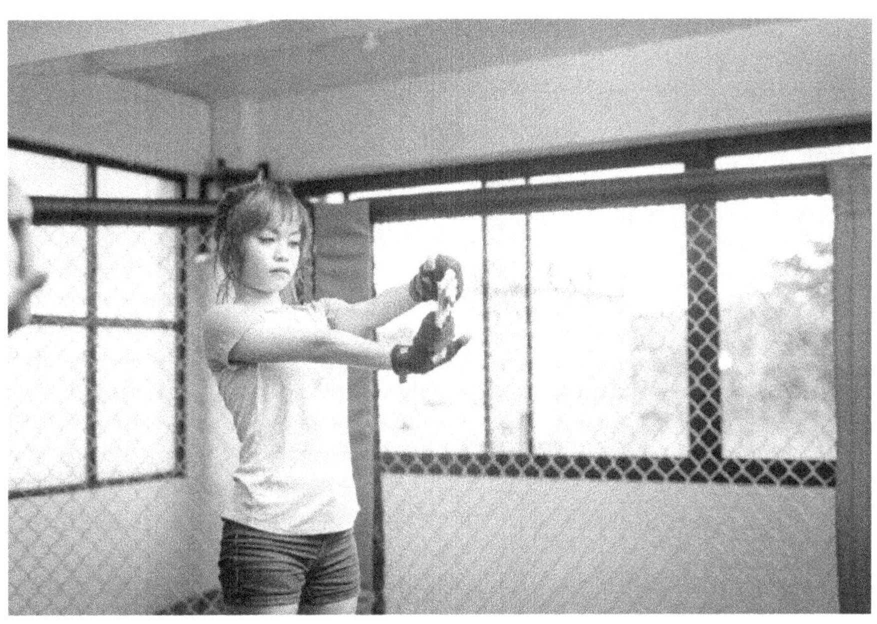

Pilates, a kind of exercise that places an emphasis on the balanced development of the body via core strength, flexibility, and awareness, has seen an enormous surge in popularity over the course of the years. In Pilates, the wand, which is sometimes referred to as the Pilates stick or bar, is one of the instruments that is utilized to enhance the efficiency of the exercises they perform. Because it provides resistance and support, the wand makes it possible for people of varying fitness levels to engage their muscles in a more efficient manner. In the following chapter, we will dig into the fundamental exercises that are utilized in wand Pilates. These exercises will include basic motions, warm-up exercises, and core-focused routines that are designed to improve strength and stability.

Basic Wand Movements and Techniques

Understand the fundamental movements and techniques involved in utilizing the Pilates wand before moving on to specialized exercises. This is an essential step before beginning particular exercises. By and large, the wand is made up of a bar that is both lightweight and flexible, and it has grips on both ends. There are a number of materials that can be used to construct it, including metal and fiberglass. By adding the wand into standard Pilates movements, the intention is to increase the level of difficulty and resistance that is used.

1. Holding the wand with an overhand grip and placing your hands shoulder-width apart is the first step in the manipulation process. Always keep your spine in a neutral position and stand with your feet hip-width apart. Maintaining stability during the workouts requires that you engage the muscles in your core.

2. Range of Motion: While completing wand exercises, you should take the time to explore the whole range of motion. The wand must be moved throughout its entire length without compromising its form in order to accomplish this endeavor. Both flexibility and joint mobility are improved as a result of this effort.

3. Breathing: Just like in regular Pilates, it is crucial to breathe correctly during this exercise. Inhale deeply through the nose, which will cause the ribcage to expand, and exhale completely through the lips that are pursed. Facilitating the mind-body connection and increasing the overall effectiveness of the exercises can be accomplished by coordinating breath with movement.

4. Moves That Are Controlled: Pay attention to motions that are controlled and deliberate. In order to successfully finish the exercises, you should avoid relying

on momentum or the flexibility of the wand. The engagement of muscles is emphasized, and general body awareness is improved as a result.

In light of the fact that we have a solid basis in wand techniques, let's investigate some warm-up exercises that will get the body ready for more difficult Pilates routines.

Warm-up Exercises with the Wand

Increasing the amount of blood that flows to the muscles, improving flexibility, and lowering the risk of injury are all achieved through the process of warming up, which is an essential component of any workout regimen. An additional level of difficulty and involvement can be added to the warm-up exercises by incorporating the Pilates wand into the routine.

1. Holding the wand with both hands and extending your arms in front of you, perform the wand arm circles exercise. Using the wand, start generating little circles in a clockwise pattern by moving it around. Slowly increase the size of the circle while concentrating on improving shoulder mobility. When the allotted time has passed, move to circles that are counterclockwise. Warming up the shoulders and upper back is the purpose of this workout.

2. By standing with your feet hip-width apart and holding the wand overhead with both hands, you can perform a side bend with the wand. By taking a deep breath in and then slightly leaning to one side as you exhale, you will be able to create a lateral stretch along the torso. Repeat on the opposite side, then inhale back to the center of the body. This not only develops flexibility but also warms up the muscles on the side.

3. When performing squats with a wand, position the wand so that it is parallel to your shoulders and behind your upper back. Hold the wand with both hands— one at each end. Place your feet slightly wider than hip-width apart while you are standing. Inhale as you lower yourself into a squat position, making sure that your knees are in line with your toes. As you return to the beginning posture, let out a long exhalation. At the same time as it activates the core, this warms up the lower body.

4. For the rotation twists of the wand, hold it in front of you with both hands and extend your arms out in front of you. Your hips should be facing forward while you rotate your torso to one side throughout this exercise. To return to the center, take a deep breath in while you twist, and then exhale. Repeat the process on the opposite side. The spine is warmed up and rotational mobility is improved with the use of this exercise.

Core Wand Exercises for Strength and Stability

1. **Wand Roll-Ups:** Assume a supine position with your legs stretched out and the wand raised above your head. Take a deep breath in, and as you exhale, squeeze your abdominal muscles to lift the wand and roll yourself up into a seated position. To roll back down with control, inhale at the height of the movement, and then exhale. This workout targets the entire core and places an emphasis on strengthening the abdominal muscles.

2. **Wand Plank Rows:** Make sure that the wand is under your hands and that it is parallel to your shoulders when you begin in the plank posture. Maintain a firm grip on the wand with one hand and move it in the direction of your hip to activate

the lat muscles. In order to exchange sides, return to the plank posture. This exercise presents a challenge to the core and works on strengthening the unilateral muscles.

3. **Wand Teasers:** Assume a supine position with your legs stretched out and the wand raised above your head. In order to get ready, take a deep breath in and as you exhale, lift both your legs and the wand at the same time, reaching all the way down to your toes. With a controlled inhalation, lower yourself back down. A high level of coordination is required for this challenging workout, which emphasizes the entire core.

4. **Wand Side Planks:** Start by holding the wand above your head while you are in a side plank posture. As you move from your head to your heels, keep a straight line. Take a big breath in, and as you feel yourself exhaling, bring the wand down under your body and reach it toward the ground. To get back to the beginning position, take a deep breath. In addition to strengthening the obliques, this exercise also helps improve lateral stability.

5. **Wand Hundred:** While lying on your back, place your legs so that they are in a tabletop posture. Hold the wand above your chest. As you exhale for a count of five, pump the wand up and down. Inhale for a count of five, and then exhale for a count of five. This pattern should be repeated for a total of one hundred pumps. The Wand Hundred is a well-known Pilates exercise that focuses on the entire abdominal region and incorporates regulated breathing.

It is possible to substantially improve your strength, stability, and total body awareness by incorporating six core wand Pilates movements into your regimen. It is important to keep in mind that you should begin with the fundamental movements and then progressively transition to more advanced workouts as your strength and overall skill improve. In addition, it is important to continually pay attention to your body and make adjustments to the exercises if you feel any discomfort or pain. If you check with a fitness professional or a healthcare provider, you should also change the exercises.

Chapter 4:

Advanced Wand Pilates Exercises

Pilates, which places an emphasis on core strength, flexibility, and overall body awareness, has been a well-liked type of exercise for a very long time. Over the past few years, there has been a growing interest in introducing a variety of props into the Pilates regimen in order to improve the overall experience. Among these props, the wand is one that has garnered attention due to the versatility and efficacy it possesses.

We are going to dig into the world of advanced wand Pilates exercises in this chapter. We are going to investigate the transition from fundamental movements to hard full-body workouts. Practitioners of Pilates can take their practice to the next level by introducing the wand into their usual routines. This will bring a new depth to their strength and flexibility training.

Progressing from Basic to Advanced Wand Exercises

First, it is essential to lay a strong foundation with fundamental wand movements before moving on to more complex exercises. By performing these fundamental exercises, practitioners are able to build the requisite coordination, balance, and body awareness that are required for more complex routines.

1. Wand Stability Drill:

One of the most important aspects of Pilates is stability, which is frequently difficult for beginners to maintain. In order to improve core strength and balance, the wand stability practice is particularly effective. As you begin, position yourself so that your feet are hip-width apart and hold the wand in front of you in a horizontal position with both hands. Keeping the wand parallel to the ground, slowly elevate one leg off the ground and move the knee closer to your chest. Do this while maintaining the position of the wand. When you have finished holding for a few seconds, switch legs. The core muscles are challenged by this exercise, which also helps to improve stability.

2. Wand Rotation with Squats:

The wand rotation with squats is a dynamic addition to the standard stability drill, which is built upon the foundation of the drill. With your elbows bent, hold the wand in front of your chest in a vertical position. Begin by performing a squat while rotating the wand to one side. After returning to the center of the body, perform another squat while rotating the wand to the opposite side. This exercise works the abdominal muscles, the legs, and the upper body all at the same time, which helps to build functional strength.

3. Single-Leg Wand Deadlift:

While also testing your balance and coordination, the single-leg wand deadlift is a great exercise for targeting your hamstrings, glutes, and lower back. Keeping both hands in front of you with the palms facing your body, hold the wand in your hands. You should flex at the hips and lift one leg behind you while simultaneously lowering the wand towards the ground. Keep the back straight and come back to the place you were in when you started. Not only does this exercise improve proprioception, but it also helps strengthen the posterior chain when performed correctly.

4. Plank with Wand Reach:

By elevating the plank position to a higher elevation, the plank with wand reach posture presents an additional challenge to the upper body. The wand should be held in one hand while you begin in the plank position. After bringing the arm that is holding the wand parallel to the ground, extend it forward and then return to the plank position from where you started. Alternate hands and say it again. The abdominal muscles, the shoulders, and the muscles that stabilize the body are all worked more intensely during this exercise.

5. Wand Teaser:

The wand teaser is a version of the traditional Pilates teaser that uses the prop with the purpose of providing additional resistance. Get into a supine position with your legs up and the wand held above your head. Lift the wand toward the ceiling as you roll yourself up into a seated position. This will create a straight line from your fingertips to your toes. Roll back down to the starting position in a slow and steady manner. The entire core is put to the test in this challenging workout, which also provides an increase in spinal flexibility.

Incorporating the Wand into Traditional Pilates Routines

After the practitioners have achieved a level of mastery in the fundamental wand movements, it is time to incorporate the prop into the conventional Pilates routines in a seamless manner. This not only makes the workouts more interesting but also increases the amount of different muscle groups that are being worked out concurrently.

1. Reformer Exercises with the Wand:

For individuals who are already familiar with the Pilates reformer, the addition of the wand might provide a new depth to the exercises that are traditionally performed. During the footwork sequence, for instance, practitioners might challenge their stability and core engagement by holding the wand overhead or across their chest with the intention of exercising their core. By the same token, including the wand into leg circles or the frog exercise performed on the reformer results in an increase in resistance and necessitates a higher level of control.

2. Mat Pilates with the Wand:

Mat Those who are passionate about Pilates can take their practice to the next level by incorporating the wand into their regular routines. During the hundred exercise, for instance, you should lift the wand off the mat while simultaneously pumping your arms. You should grasp the wand in both hands. Not only does this make the effort for the abdominal muscles more difficult, but it also utilizes the shoulders and arms more significantly. To improve your stability and balance while performing the side plank, position the wand such that it runs along your bottom arm.

3. Cadillac and Tower Exercises:

Both the Cadillac and the Tower equipment include a number of different attachment points for the wand, which enables a large variety of workouts to be performed. As an illustration, the lower body is challenged in novel ways when the wand is used in conjunction with leg springs during the leg circles or leg springs series. There is also the possibility of incorporating the wand into arm workouts performed on the Tower, which will result in increased resistance and improved alignment.

4. Magic Circle and Wand Fusion:

By combining the magic circle and the wand, a dynamic fusion is created that simultaneously addresses the upper body as well as the lower body. To illustrate, when you are seated, you should position the magic circle so that it is between your ankles and hold the wand over your head. During the process of applying pressure to the magic circle, lift your legs off the ground and bring the wand closer to the ground. This will engage your core as well as your inner thighs.

Challenging Full-Body Workouts with the Wand

Practitioners are able to engage on rigorous full-body routines that stretch their limits and develop their overall strength and flexibility when they have a good foundation in basic and intermediate wand movements.

1. Wand Circuit Training:

Develop a circuit that includes a variety of wand movements, making sure to segue from one movement to the next in a smooth and fluid manner. To give you an example, begin with squats with a wand, then go on to lunges with a wand, and then finish with wand rotations with planks. A cardiovascular component, as well as benefits for strength and flexibility, are provided by this circuit, which challenges the complete body while also giving benefits.

2. Dynamic Wand Flow:

Using the wand, you should develop a flowing sequence of movements that allows you to segue from one exercise to the next without any interruptions. For example, you could start with wand stability drills, then transition into wand rotations with squats, and finally go on to single-leg wand deadlifts. By maintaining the muscles engaged for the entirety of the workout, this dynamic flow helps to improve both endurance and coordination.

3. Advanced Wand Pilates Routine:

Build a full Pilates practice that includes more complex exercises using a wand technique. Begin with a warm-up that consists of fundamental wand motions, and then progressively go on to exercises that are more difficult. It is important to target different muscle groups, hence it is important to include a range of positions, such as standing, sitting, and lying down. This advanced practice can be tailored to the specific fitness levels of each individual, allowing for growth over the course of repeated sessions.

4. Partner Wand Workouts:

Utilize the wand to perform workouts with a partner in order to increase motivation and promote responsibility. Resistance training, balance drills, and dynamic movements are all examples of workouts that can be performed with a partner. One partner, for instance, may hold the wand in a horizontal position while the other partner performs squats. This would result in the creation of resistance and would also put an aspect of collaboration into the workout.

For Pilates practitioners who are looking to improve their strength, flexibility, and overall fitness, the use of the wand into more advanced Pilates movements opens up new possibilities. The wand is a versatile and effective prop that can be used for a variety of purposes, beginning with the progression of basic movements and progressing to the seamless incorporation of the wand into traditional Pilates routines, and ultimately leading to the completion of challenging full-body workouts. It is essential to pay attention to your body, make progress at your own pace, and seek the advice of a fitness professional or a healthcare provider if necessary. This is one of the most important aspects of any workout program. Through the use of the principles of Pilates, the advanced wand Pilates exercises that are taught in this chapter offer a way to achieve ongoing improvement and a more profound connection with one's own body.

Chapter 5:

Targeted Muscle Groups

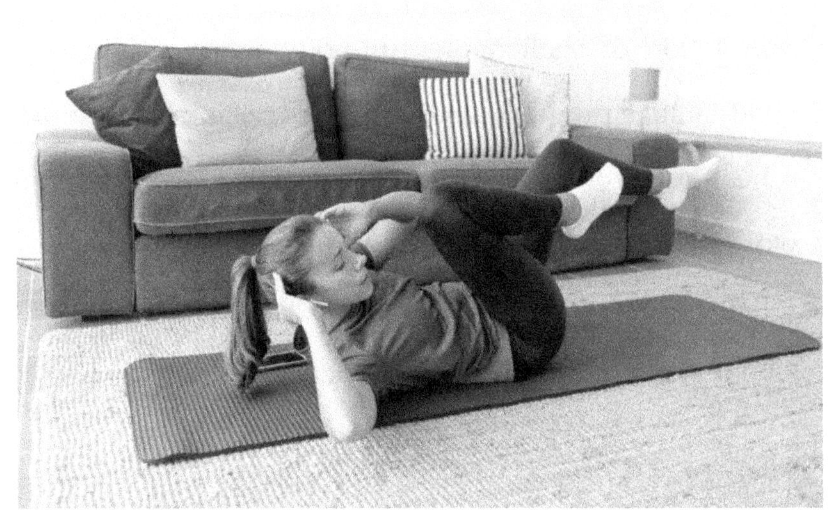

Within the realm of physical fitness, having a solid understanding of how to target particular muscle groups is absolutely necessary in order to achieve a comprehensive level of strength, flexibility, and total body balance. This chapter examines specific exercises that are designed to engage and build distinct muscle groups. It also provides insights on how to tailor workouts to specific fitness goals. Incorporating specific workouts into your regimen can lead to more effective and efficient outcomes, regardless of whether your goal is to tone the core, sculpt the arms, or improve leg strength.

Core Muscles:

The core is the most powerful part of the body because it provides the body with stability and support for a variety of muscle actions. When it comes to improvement of posture, balance, and total functional fitness, targeting the core is absolutely necessary.

1. Plank Variations:

Planks are an essential exercise for working out the entire core at once. By using variants like as side planks, plank twists, and plank with leg lifts, you may strengthen the focus on other muscles and make the workout more challenging. The obliques, transverse abdominis, and rectus abdominis are all activated with these variations, which contribute to an overall increase in core strength.

2. Bicycle Crunches:

Bicycle crunches are a dynamic workout that engage the rectus abdominis as well as the obliques when performed correctly. While lying on your back, elevate your legs off the ground and bring your opposing elbow to your opposite knee in a cycling motion. Repeat this motion for the other side. This exercise strengthens coordination while targeting the entire abdominal region that is being worked.

3. Russian Twists:

Execute Russian twists by twisting your torso from side to side while seated or reclined on the floor. You may also perform this exercise while holding a weight or medicine ball. Rotational strength is crucial for a wide variety of activities and sports, and this exercise helps develop rotational strength by engaging the obliques.

4. Boat Pose:

To work the entire core, incorporate yoga-inspired poses such as the Boat Pose into your routine. Place your feet flat on the ground, lean back, elevate your legs, and extend your arms in front of you. The rectus abdominis is the muscle that is targeted by this exercise, which also strengthens the link between your core muscles.

Arms and Shoulders:

Developing arms that are both strong and toned improves functional strength and provides assistance for day-to-day activities. The following workouts are specifically designed to target the biceps, triceps, and shoulders.

1. Bicep Curls:

Use dumbbells or resistance bands for bicep curls. Stand with feet hip-width apart, and lift the weights towards your shoulders while keeping your elbows close to your body. This exercise isolates the biceps and promotes arm strength.

2. Tricep Dips:

Position your hands on a stable surface behind you, fingers facing forward. Lower your body by bending your elbows, then push back up. Tricep dips effectively target the triceps and improve arm definition.

3. Shoulder Press:

Hold dumbbells at shoulder height with palms facing forward. Press the weights overhead, extending your arms fully. Shoulder presses target the deltoids, strengthening the shoulders and upper arms.

4. Push-ups:

Classic push-ups engage multiple muscle groups, including the chest, triceps, and shoulders. Modify the intensity by adjusting hand placement or incorporating variations like diamond push-ups or decline push-ups.

Legs and Glutes:

Building strength in the lower body is vital for overall mobility, stability, and athleticism. Target the quads, hamstrings, and glutes with these exercises.

1. Squats:

Squats are a foundational leg exercise. Stand with feet shoulder-width apart and lower your body by bending your knees. Squats engage the quadriceps, hamstrings, and glutes, promoting overall lower body strength.

2. Lunges:

Forward lunges, reverse lunges, and lateral lunges target different muscles in the legs and glutes. Step forward, backward, or to the side, bending your knees and keeping your upper body upright to maximize engagement.

3. Deadlifts:

Deadlifts target the hamstrings, glutes, and lower back. Whether using a barbell or dumbbells, hinge at the hips while keeping the back straight, lowering the weights towards the ground, and then returning to a standing position.

4. Calf Raises:

Strengthen the calf muscles by performing calf raises. Stand on a flat surface and lift your heels off the ground, rising onto the balls of your feet. This exercise targets the gastrocnemius and soleus muscles.

Back Muscles:

A strong back contributes to good posture, spine health, and overall upper body strength. Incorporate these exercises to target the latissimus dorsi, rhomboids, and erector spinae.

1. Lat Pulldowns:

Using a cable machine or resistance band, perform lat pulldowns to target the latissimus dorsi. Pull the bar or band down towards your chest while keeping your back straight.

2. Bent-Over Rows:

Hold dumbbells in each hand, hinge at the hips, and row the weights towards your hips. Bent-over rows engage the rhomboids and upper back muscles.

3. Superman Exercise:

Lie face down on the floor, lift your arms and legs off the ground simultaneously, engaging the erector spinae along the spine. The Superman exercise helps strengthen the muscles of the lower back.

4. Reverse Flyes:

Using dumbbells, bend forward at the hips, and lift the weights to the sides while keeping your arms straight. Reverse flyes target the rear deltoids and upper back muscles.

Tailoring Workouts for Specific Fitness Goals:

Understanding how to tailor workouts based on individual fitness goals is essential for achieving desired results. Whether the aim is weight loss, muscle gain, or improved endurance, customization is key.

1. Weight Loss:

A combination of cardiovascular workouts and strength training that targets the entire body is an excellent training regimen for individuals who are trying to lose excess weight. Through the utilization of exercises that activate numerous muscle groups, high-intensity interval training (HIIT) sessions are able to facilitate the burning of calories and the accumulation of fat.

2. Muscle Gain:

Those who are interested in increasing their muscular mass should concentrate on performing progressive resistance exercise. It is important to place an emphasis on compound exercises like squats, deadlifts, and bench presses because these exercises target significant muscular groups. Incorporate an adequate amount of protein into your diet to assist the growth and recuperation of your muscles.

3. Endurance:

In order to improve endurance, it is necessary to combine cardiovascular training with strength exercises that involve high repetitions but low resistance during the workout. Participate in activities such as running, cycling, or swimming, and incorporate exercises that use only your own bodyweight, with only a short period of rest in between sets.

4. Flexibility and Mobility:

It is recommended that individuals who place a high priority on flexibility and mobility incorporate dynamic stretches and exercises inspired by yoga into their fitness program. In order to improve joint health and flexibility, you should focus on targeting specific muscle groups using range of motion exercises.

Tips for Targeting Specific Muscle Groups:

1. Focus on Form:

During workouts, it is important to maintain appropriate form in order to efficiently target the muscle groups that are being targeted and to reduce the risk of injury. Seek the advice of a fitness expert to ensure that you are using the appropriate approach.

2. Gradual Progression:

You should gradually increase the intensity of your workouts in order to place the muscles under increasing amounts of stress. Increasing the weights, the number of repetitions, or the complexity of the workouts can all fulfill this purpose.

3. Variety is Key:

Alternate between different workouts to prevent reaching a plateau and to ensure that your muscles are constantly being challenged. In order to target a variety of muscle groups, it is important to incorporate a combination of compound motions and isolation exercises.

4. Listen to Your Body:

You should pay attention to how your body reacts to the various activities you perform. If you are experiencing discomfort that goes beyond the normal level of muscular fatigue, you should either reevaluate your form or seek the advice of a fitness specialist.

5. Adequate Recovery:

Make sure that you give your muscles enough time to heal in between sessions. A healthy amount of rest, sufficient diet, and adequate hydration are all factors that contribute to good muscle growth and recovery.

A well-rounded fitness program should include instruction on how to target various muscle groups and how to adjust workouts to individual goals. This is an essential component of a fitness regimen. It is possible to achieve more efficient and effective outcomes by taking a targeted strategy, regardless of whether the objective is to strengthen the core, sculpt the arms, grow leg muscles, or enhance general endurance. It is essential to customize workouts according to the individual's current fitness level, preferences, and any preexisting health concerns. The goal of individuals is to obtain their desired fitness objectives and to enjoy a holistic approach to health and well-being. This can be accomplished by incorporating a range of exercises, maintaining a focus on form, and gradually progressing through the exercises.

Chapter 6:

Wand Pilates for Rehabilitation

The practice of Pilates, which is a form of exercise that emphasizes core strength, flexibility, and overall body awareness, has been increasingly popular in recent years due to the multiple health benefits that it offers. The utilization of various props, such as the wand, with the purpose of enhancing the efficiency of the exercises and catering to particular requirements is one of the unique aspects of Pilates. Within the scope of this chapter, we will investigate the utilization of wand Pilates for the purpose of rehabilitation, with a particular focus on its role in injury prevention and recovery, as well as specialized exercises specific to common injuries. In addition, we will emphasize the significance of working with medical specialists in order to develop an all-encompassing rehabilitation strategy.

Using the Wand for Injury Prevention and Recovery:

Standard Pilates movements are given an additional dimension by the use of the wand, which is a straightforward and adaptable tool. Due to the fact that its structure is elongated, it provides higher leverage and stability, making it an excellent instrument for the avoidance of injuries and the recovery from them. A Pilates routine can be properly blended with the use of the wand in the following ways:

1. Enhancing Stability and Balance: The wand can be used to enhance stability and balance during exercises that are performed using either a standing or seated position. When individuals hold the wand in a variety of positions, they engage

muscles that are responsible for stabilization, which in turn promotes improved balance and reduces the danger of falling. This is especially helpful for people who are recuperating from accidents or procedures that have been performed on their lower limbs.

2. Providing Support for Spinal Alignment It is essential to do correct spinal alignment maintenance in order to prevent injuries and to recover from them. It is possible to use the wand as a guide to ensure that perfect posture is maintained throughout specific exercises, particularly those that focus on the abdominal and back muscles. It is imperative that folks who are undergoing rehabilitation for spinal injuries or who are coping with chronic back pain follow this.

3. Increasing Range of Motion: One of the most important aspects of therapy for people who are recuperating from joint injuries or operations is progressively increasing their range of motion. In order to facilitate a safe and progressive advancement in joint flexibility, the wand can be utilized to provide assistance in performed motions that are under control. When it comes to the rehabilitation of injuries to the knee, hip, and shoulder, this is especially applicable.

4. Using the Wand to Isolate and Target Individual Muscle Groups The wand may be used to isolate and target specific muscle groups, which enables a more targeted approach to rehabilitation. Individuals are able to perform workouts that are specifically tailored to target the deficits that are linked with their particular injury by incorporating resistance and support from the wand.

Rehabilitation Exercises for Common Injuries:

The Wand Pilates program provides a wide variety of exercises that may be modified to meet the requirements of a variety of injuries and rehabilitation needs. Exercises that are specifically designed to treat common injuries are as follows:

1. **Rotator Cuff Injury – Wand Shoulder Rotations:** It is possible for individuals who are recuperating from injuries to the rotator cuff to enhance their range of motion and strengthen the muscles that surround their shoulder by performing mild shoulder rotations with the wand. The wand offers support and direction, allowing for controlled movements to be performed without putting an undue amount of effort on the shoulder that was injured.

Instructions:

- Maintain a straight posture whether you are standing or sitting.
- Maintain a firm grip on the wand with both hands, extending your arms in front of you at shoulder height.
- Concentrate on making movements that are under control and devoid of discomfort as you slowly rotate the wand to the right and then to the left.
- To complete each direction, perform ten to fifteen repetitions.

2. **Knee Injury – Wand Leg Raises:** It is common for knee injuries to necessitate specific exercises in order to reestablish strength in the quadriceps and the muscles around them. Raising the legs with a wand offers both support and resistance, which is beneficial to the rehabilitation process.

Instructions:

- The wand should be positioned horizontally under one foot while you are lying on your back.

- When you want to maintain stability, hold the ends of the wand with both hands.
- While maintaining a slight bend in the knee, lift the leg with the wand in a straight upward motion.
- The leg should be lowered back down without making contact with the ground.
- Work out between 12 and 15 repetitions on each leg.

3. **Lower Back Pain – Wand Pelvic Tilts:** Exercises that enhance pelvic stability and core strength can be beneficial for individuals who are having pain in their lower back. In addition to helping to keep the spine in a neutral position, wand pelvic tilts keep the abdominal muscles engaged.

Instructions:

- If you are lying on your back, bend your knees and place your feet flat on the ground.
- Position the wand so that it lies horizontally on top of your pelvis.
- To get ready, take a deep breath in, then exhale and lift your pelvis upward towards the wand while pressing it down.
- As you return to the starting position, take a deep breath.
- Repeat for fifteen to twenty repetitions.

4. **Ankle Sprain – Wand Ankle Circles:** A thorough rehabilitation program is necessary for restoring flexibility and strength after an ankle sprain. For the purpose of improving mobility, wand ankle circles offer a movement that is both controlled and guided.

Instructions:

- Place yourself in a seated or lying position with one leg outstretched.
- Hold the wand over the ball of the foot and move it around.
- A circular motion should be performed on the ankle while the wand is used to provide a slight resistance.
- Following the completion of ten to fifteen revolutions in each direction, switch legs.

Consultation with Healthcare Professionals for Rehabilitation:

It is vital to underline the need of working with healthcare specialists in order to develop a comprehensive and individualized strategy for recovery, despite the fact that wand Pilates has the potential to be an advantageous component of rehabilitation processes. Physical therapists, orthopedic experts, and other medical professionals play an important part in determining the severity of injuries, devising individualized rehabilitation plans, and keeping track of the patient's progress.

1. Individualized Assessment: Medical practitioners are able to carry out comprehensive evaluations in order to comprehend the nature and extent of injuries. Imaging for diagnostic purposes, tests to determine range of motion, and a thorough evaluation of the patient's medical history may all be carried out. Professionals are able to develop tailored rehabilitation plans that take into account unique requirements and constraints when they have access to this information.
2. Monitoring Progress It is vital to perform regular monitoring of progress in order

to guarantee that rehabilitation efforts are both effective and safe throughout the process. In the event that the patient has a setback or progress, medical practitioners are able to modify rehabilitation plans accordingly, making any required adjustments to the exercises and the intensity levels. It is essential to conduct this constant review in order to avoid overexertion and to ensure that optimal recuperation is achieved.

3. Coordination with Other Specialists: When there are numerous specialists participating in the care of a patient, it is essential to have excellent communication and teamwork in order to avoid any complications. Exercises performed with a wand Pilates apparatus can be used in conjunction with other forms of rehabilitation, such as chiropractic care, occupational therapy, or personal training. It is possible to achieve a holistic and integrated approach to healing through coordinated efforts.

4. Educating Patients on Home Exercises Healthcare practitioners have the ability to educate patients on the correct way to perform basic Pilates exercises as part of their home rehabilitation regimen. The empowerment of individuals to take an active role in their own recovery can be facilitated by the provision of clear instructions, demonstrations, and feedback on form and technique. Moreover, this knowledge encourages commitment to the workouts that have been suggested.

5. Rehabilitation is not only a physical process; it also incorporates psychological aspects such as motivation, resilience, and mental well-being. It is important to address these psychological aspects of rehabilitation. Healthcare personnel are able to offer support and assistance, addressing any emotional issues or concerns that may occur during the course of the rehabilitation process. An strategy that takes a comprehensive perspective helps to contribute to a more happy and

effective rehabilitation.

Wand The Pilates method is a versatile and useful tool for rehabilitation, as it provides exercises that are specifically designed to assist in the prevention of injuries and the recovery from them. Individuals are able to improve their stability, increase their range of motion, and target specific muscle groups that are crucial for recovery when they incorporate the wand into their Pilates exercises. Nevertheless, it is of the utmost importance to acknowledge the significance of consulting with healthcare specialists in order to develop a therapeutic strategy that is both thorough and individualized. Assessment of injuries, creation of specific rehabilitation plans, and monitoring of progress are all important responsibilities that fall under the purview of physical therapists and other practitioners. The utilization of wand Pilates in conjunction with the instruction of a trained expert results in a synergistic approach to rehabilitation that fosters optimal recovery and long-term well-being throughout time.

Chapter 7:

Wand Pilates for Special Populations

In order to cater to the specific requirements of special populations, Wand Pilates, which is a form of exercise that is both gentle and effective, can be modified. In this chapter, we dig into the methods in which workouts can be altered for those who have physical limitations, address the considerations for wand Pilates during pregnancy and postpartum, and investigate modified exercises that are specifically designed for older citizens. Everyone, regardless of age, stage of life, or physical condition, should be able to participate in Pilates and reap the benefits of doing so. This is the primary objective.

Modified Exercises for Seniors:

As people get older, their bodies go through a number of changes that can have an effect on their capacity to participate in particular types of physical activities. Pilates with a Wand is a fantastic choice for senior citizens since it is a low-impact, joint-friendly method that helps improve strength, flexibility, and balance. It is essential to make modifications in order to guarantee that senior citizens may reap the benefits of Pilates while taking into account the specific challenges they face.

1. Seated Wand Exercises:

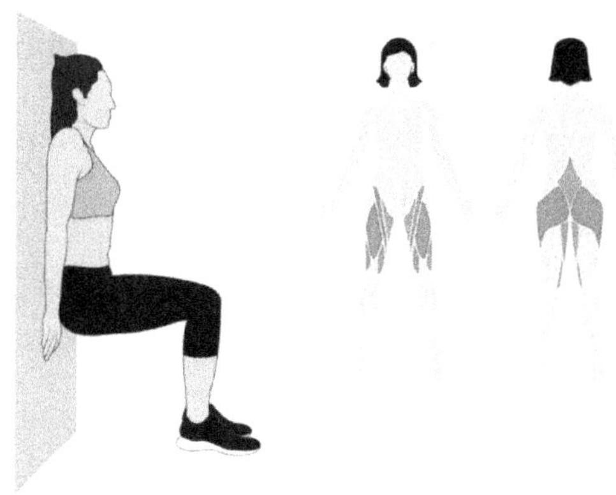

Seated wand exercises have the potential to be very useful for senior citizens who have mobility limitations or who suffer from discomfort when performing standing activities. When used in a seated position, the wand can be utilized as a tool to improve flexibility and engage the core muscles. Incorporating gentle twists, side bends, and forward stretches into your routine will help alleviate stiffness and promote spinal mobility.

2. Chair-Assisted Exercises:

Seniors might utilize a chair as a prop while performing wand Pilates movements in order to provide themselves with more support. Individuals are able to concentrate on controlled motions without the worry of falling because the chair provides assistance with balance and stability. The wand can be used to perform seated leg lifts, arm exercises, and torso rotations, all of which can be easily included into a routine that employs chair assistance.

3. Slow and Controlled Movements:

Movements performed at a slower rate during regular Pilates sessions may be beneficial for senior citizens. Through the use of this careful approach, one is able to cultivate mindfulness and reduce the likelihood of harm while simultaneously increasing their awareness of each motion. A further benefit of putting an emphasis on controlled motions is that it helps to increase muscle strength and endurance over time.

4. Customizing Resistance Levels:

There is a wide range of resistance levels available for wands, and it is beneficial for elderly citizens to select a wand that corresponds with their current level of strength and fitness. It is possible to customize resistance to ensure that the workouts continue to be tough while also being attainable. This allows for progressive improvement without generating undue strain.

Pregnancy and Postpartum Wand Pilates:

Due to the fact that pregnancy and the postpartum period are both transforming seasons in a woman's life, it is important to exercise with caution during these times. In the event that adaptations are made to fit the physiological changes and specific requirements of pregnant and new mothers, wand Pilates has the potential to be a treatment option that is both safe and effective.

1. Core Engagement with Caution:

In order to safeguard the developing baby and accommodate the changes that occur in the mother's body, it is necessary to make adjustments to the standard Pilates exercises that are performed during pregnancy. Wand Pilates can be used as an alternative to traditional crunches by concentrating on mild core engagement through pelvic tilts, pelvic floor exercises, and modified abdominal work. This helps to maintain strength without subjecting the body to strain.

2. Emphasizing Postural Alignment:

It is common for a woman's center of gravity to shift during pregnancy, which can result in alterations to her posture and balance. By putting an emphasis on movements that improve postural alignment, Wand Pilates can be helpful in addressing these concerns. Exercising the spine gently, rolling the shoulders, and tilting the pelvis are all examples of exercises that can help alleviate discomfort and preserve healthy posture.

3. Pelvic Floor Exercises:

In light of the fact that the pelvic floor is of utmost significance during pregnancy and postpartum recovery, wand Pilates may be adapted to include particular movements that focus on this region. The pelvic floor muscles are strengthened by the use of these exercises, which contributes to improved bladder control and postpartum recovery outcomes.

4. Gradual Progression Postpartum:

When it comes to assisting new mothers in gradually regaining strength and tone in their abdominal and pelvic muscles after giving birth, wand Pilates can be an extremely helpful tool. During the first few weeks after giving birth, it is critical to move carefully, to adhere to the natural healing process of the body, and to refrain from engaging in activities that involve high-impact motions.

Adapting Workouts for Individuals with Physical Limitations:

It is well known that Pilates is adaptable, which means that it is suited for people who have a variety of physical restrictions or disabilities. In order to cater to the specific requirements of individuals who are dealing with physical obstacles, Pilates can be adapted through the modification of exercises and the utilization of various props, including wands.

1. Seated and Supine Positions:

When it comes to those who have restricted movement or who are unable to stand, seated and supine positions become quite necessary. In order to ensure that participants are able to engage in a full-body workout while remaining sitting or lying down in a comfortable position, Wand Pilates movements can be adapted to these situations.

2. Joint-Friendly Movements:

Due to the low-impact nature of wand Pilates, it may be considered good for individuals who suffer from illnesses such as arthritis, joint discomfort, or other musculoskeletal ailments. The prevention of an exacerbation of pain while simultaneously improving strength and flexibility can be accomplished by avoiding high-impact exercises and introducing motions that are pleasant to the joints.

3. Mindful Breathing Techniques:

Pilates is a form of exercise that lays a significant emphasis on mindful breathing, which is especially good for people who have respiratory issues or reduced lung capacity. It is possible to modify Wand Pilates such that it incorporates breathing exercises that improve lung function and induce relaxation, so contributing to a general improvement in well-being.

4. Personalized Modifications:

Because the physical constraints of each person are different, it is essential to make changes that are individualized in order to make Pilates accessible to everyone. Instructors who work with clients who have physical challenges should have a comprehensive awareness of the individual needs of their clients and should modify exercises to meet those needs. This will ensure that the practice is both safe and effective.

Because of its adaptability and variety, Wand Pilates has shown to be a fitness method that is both inclusive and accessible to individuals who belong to particular demographics. Pilates can be adapted to fit the varied requirements of practitioners by altering exercises for senior citizens, addressing the specific concerns that arise during pregnancy and postpartum, and adapting routines for persons who have physical restrictions. In order to ensure that everyone, regardless of age or physical condition, is able to experience the multiple benefits that wand Pilates has to offer, this chapter emphasizes the significance of customization, mindfulness, and progressive growth.

Chapter 8:

Incorporating Props and Accessories

Workouts in the realm of Pilates can be given a new dimension via the utilization of various props and accessories, which can enhance both the diversity and the efficiency of the workouts. Within the scope of Chapter 8, the creative integration of props is investigated, with a particular emphasis placed on integrating the wand with various additional Pilates accessories. The practitioners are able to construct dynamic and varied workouts that target multiple muscle groups, improve flexibility, and boost overall balance when they do this.

Combining the Wand with Other Pilates Props:

1. **Resistance Bands:**
   - **Purpose:** Combining the wand with resistance bands adds an extra element of resistance to exercises, intensifying muscle engagement.
   - **Examples:** Wrap a resistance band around the wand and perform arm exercises, such as lateral raises or bicep curls, to target the upper body with increased resistance.

2. **Pilates Rings (Magic Circles):**

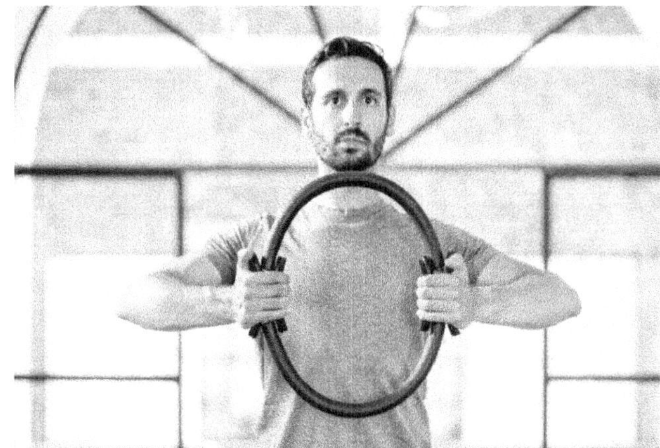

- **Purpose:** The Pilates ring can be used in conjunction with the wand to provide targeted resistance for both the upper and lower body.
- **Examples:** Place the Pilates ring between the ankles and use the wand for stability during leg lifts, creating a challenging workout for the inner and outer thighs.

3. **Exercise Balls:**

- **Purpose:** Incorporating an exercise ball adds an element of instability, engaging the core muscles and promoting balance.
- **Examples:** Sit on the exercise ball with the wand overhead, performing controlled upper body movements to challenge stability and core strength.

4. **Foam Rollers:**

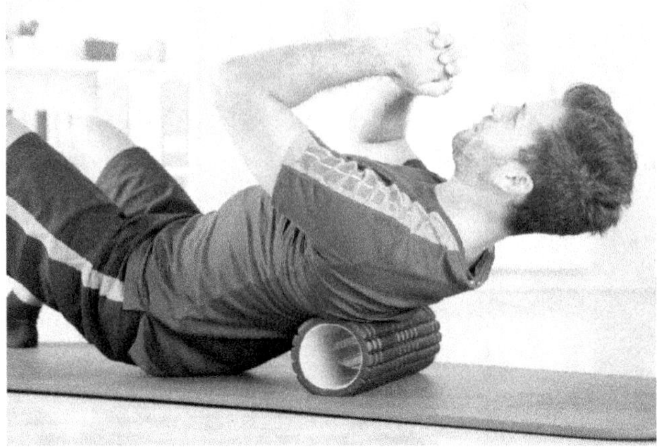

- **Purpose:** Utilizing a foam roller can enhance proprioception and balance while providing a gentle massage effect.
- **Examples:** Perform wand exercises while balancing on a foam roller, engaging stabilizing muscles for a more comprehensive workout.

Creating Dynamic and Varied Workouts:

1. **Circuit Training:**

- **Purpose:** Designing circuit-style workouts with the wand and various props keeps sessions dynamic and prevents monotony.
- **Examples:** Rotate through different exercises using the wand, resistance bands, Pilates rings, and other props in a timed sequence to maintain interest and challenge the body.

2. **Interval Training:**

- **Purpose:** Alternating between periods of high and low intensity using different props helps improve cardiovascular fitness while targeting different muscle groups.

- **Examples:** Integrate wand exercises with high-intensity bursts using resistance bands or Pilates rings, followed by a recovery period with low-impact movements.

3. **Functional Movement Patterns:**

- **Purpose:** Incorporate functional movements that mimic daily activities to enhance overall mobility and strength.
- **Examples:** Use the wand in combination with a stability ball for squats or lunges, promoting functional strength and balance.

4. **Progressive Sequences:**

- **Purpose:** Gradually increase the complexity of exercises within a single session to challenge participants and encourage continual improvement.
- **Examples:** Begin with basic wand exercises and progressively add in different props, increasing the difficulty as participants build strength and confidence.

Enhancing Flexibility and Balance with Additional Accessories:

1. **Stretch Bands:**

- **Purpose:** Adding stretch bands to wand Pilates enhances flexibility by providing gentle resistance during stretches.
- **Examples:** Use the wand for stability while incorporating stretch bands into various stretches, promoting increased flexibility in the shoulders, hips, and spine.

2. **Balance Pads:**

- **Purpose:** Enhancing balance is crucial for overall stability and injury prevention. Balance pads can be integrated into wand exercises for an added challenge.

- **Examples:** Stand on a balance pad while performing wand exercises to engage stabilizing muscles and improve balance.

3. **Ankle Weights:**

- **Purpose:** Ankle weights can be strategically incorporated to increase the intensity of lower body exercises, promoting strength and stability.
- **Examples:** Strap on ankle weights while performing leg lifts with the wand to target the quadriceps and hamstrings effectively.

4. **Yoga Blocks:**

- **Purpose:** Yoga blocks can be used to modify exercises and accommodate different levels of flexibility.
- **Examples:** During seated stretches with the wand, place yoga blocks under the hands to provide support and allow participants to gradually progress into deeper stretches.

Adding accessories and props to the wand through incorporation Not only does Pilates increase the variety of exercises that are performed, but it also makes the exercises more effective as a whole. By utilizing the wand in conjunction with many other Pilates props, it is possible to create sessions that are both creative and dynamic, focusing on different muscle groups and areas of fitness. Practise that incorporates props keeps participants interested while continuously challenging and developing their strength, flexibility, and balance. This can be accomplished through circuit training, interval training, functional movement patterns, or progressive sequences. This chapter demonstrates the numerous possibilities for designing entertaining and well-rounded workouts through the creative use of props and accessories, and it emphasizes the versatility of wand Pilates as a form of exercise.

Chapter 9:

Mind-Body Connection in Wand Pilates

In addition to the physical aspects of fitness, Wand Pilates, which is a form of exercise that incorporates the use of a wand or a pole, also expands beyond those characteristics. The book dives into the complex interaction that exists between the mind and the body, putting an emphasis on the significance of breathing, mindfulness, and the connection between the mind and the body. Over the course of this chapter, we will investigate how Wand Pilates offers a distinctive method of physical activity by embracing these concepts and the mental advantages that it provides..

Focusing on Breath and Mindfulness:

One of the characteristics that sets Wand Pilates apart from other forms of Pilates is the emphasis placed on mindful breathing and conscious breathing. Wand Pilates places the breath at the center of each and every movement, in contrast to more conventional types of exercise, which may take the breath for granted. A harmonious flow that involves both the mind and the body can be created with the help of the wand, which functions as a tool to synchronize the breath with specific motions.

Practitioners of Wand Pilates are strongly urged to concentrate on the quality of their breath for the entirety of the instruction session. The individual is guided to establish a profound connection with their breath through the inhalation and exhalation aspects of each movement, which become important parts of the movement structure. The conscious attention that is paid to the breath not only makes the exercises more effective, but it also acts as a gateway to the practice of mindfulness.

Being totally present and engaged in the moment is what is meant by the term "mindfulness" when used to the setting of Wand Pilates. The individuals acquire a heightened awareness of their bodies as they devote their attention to the sensations of their breath and the movements of the wand within their bodies. Beyond the confines of the training session, this mindfulness practice encourages a sense of presence in the routines of daily life and helps to cultivate a more profound connection between the mind and the body.

Incorporating Principles of Mind-Body Connection:

The mind-body connection is a fundamental aspect of Wand Pilates. The use of the wand acts as a conduit for this connection, bridging the gap between mental focus and physical execution. Several principles contribute to the integration of the mind and body in Wand Pilates:

1. Concentration: In order to execute exercises with accuracy, Wand Pilates calls for a degree of concentration that is exceptionally high. In order to get optimal results, the practitioner will pay their attention to the alignment of the body, the positioning of the wand, and the coordination of the breath. Not only does this increased concentration help to enhance the physical exercise, but it also helps to engage the mind in a meditative state.
2. The Pilates philosophy places a significant emphasis on the concept of the "powerhouse," which refers to the core muscles that are responsible for providing both stability and strength. The practice of Wand Pilates involves a significant

emphasis on centering, which encourages participants to activate and engage their core throughout the performance of the movements. This not only helps to strengthen the physical core, but it also helps to promote a sense of emotional stability and a sense of being grounded.

3. Flow: The fluidity of movement in Wand Pilates helps to contribute to the connection between the mind and the body. Individuals are able to experience a continuous flow that needs mental concentration and physical coordination as they transition from one activity to another in a smooth manner. This state of flow fosters a sense of unity between the mind and the body, which contributes to an overall improvement in well-being.

4. Body Awareness: Wand Pilates helps individuals become more aware of their bodies by training them to pay attention to seemingly insignificant movements, the engagement of their muscles, and the alignment of their bodies. As practitioners gradually develop a greater awareness of their bodies, they also develop a more profound comprehension of the ways in which their mental concentration affects their physical performance.

The Mental Benefits of Wand Pilates:

Wand Pilates provides a multitude of mental benefits that help to general well-being, in addition to the physical changes that are connected with regular exercise. These advantages are not limited to the time spent in a Pilates session; rather, they have an impact on other aspects of life as well as mental toughness. Among the many mental advantages of Wand Pilates are the following:

1. Reducing Stress: The mix of attentive breathing, regulated movements, and aware

breathing that is used in Wand Pilates produces a setting that is beneficial to reducing stress. Individuals are able to release stress, both physically and psychologically, through the practice of mindful Pilates, which in turn promotes a sense of serenity and relaxation.

2. Enhancement of Concentration and Focus: The concentration that is required in Wand Pilates not only contributes to the efficiency of the exercises, but it also translates to an improvement in concentration when performing activities that are part of daily life. Pilates practitioners frequently claim enhanced attention and mental clarity, attributing these benefits to the disciplined mental attitude that is developed via consistent Pilates practice.

3. Wand Pilates encourages a heightened awareness of the body and the movements that it moves through, which results in enhanced mind-body awareness. This increased sensitivity to bodily sensations extends to an awareness of mental and emotional states as well as mental and emotional states. There is a possibility that individuals will become more aware of their own ideas and emotions, which will present them with an opportunity for introspection and personal development.

4. The attentive approach to movement that is utilized in Wand Pilates is designed to provide a positive contribution to the mental well-being of its participants. People are able to experience a sort of moving meditation by establishing a connection between their breath and their movements and by being totally present in each practice. It is possible to use this mindful movement as a therapeutic practice, which will help to promote mental resilience and emotional equilibrium.

5. The Wand Pilates method places an emphasis on functional movement and the development of a strong, flexible, and balanced body. This results in an increase in body positivity. When people see advances in their physical capabilities, they

frequently experience a favorable shift in their image of their bodies. This enhanced body positivity has the potential to have a significant influence on both one's sense of self-worth and their mental health.

6. Mind-Body Harmony: The incorporation of breath, mindfulness, and the mind-body connection into Wand Pilates helps to cultivate a feeling of harmony between the mental and physical components of the individual. The effects of this harmony extend beyond the confines of the workout, affecting how individuals respond to obstacles, how they choose to proceed, and how they handle the intricacies of everyday life.

In Chapter 9, we discussed the importance of the mind-body connection in Wand Pilates. Some of the topics that were covered included the relevance of breath, mindfulness, and the integration of mental and physical concepts. Through the provision of a holistic approach that nurtures both the body and the mind, Wand Pilates goes beyond the conventional methods of physical training.

Individuals are able to not only develop their physical strength and flexibility, but also cultivate their mental resilience and well-being via the use of a one-of-a-kind training experience that is defined by the focus placed on breathing and mindfulness. A profound mind-body connection is created through the application of the principles of concentration, centering, flow, and body awareness, which together create a practice that transcends beyond the confines of the studio and into aspects of everyday life.

Wand Pilates is a valuable addition to one's holistic health and wellness routine because of the mental benefits it offers, which include the reduction of stress, the improvement of concentration, the enhancement of mind-body awareness, mindful movement for mental well-being, increased body positivity, and overall mind-body harmony. In the process of adopting the mindful approach of Wand Pilates, individuals discover a road that leads not just to improved physical fitness but also to a life that is more balanced and brought into focus.

Chapter 10:

Wand Pilates and Nutrition

The holistic approach that is utilized in Wand Pilates goes beyond the sphere of physical activity and encompasses a variety of factors of well-being, including an emphasis on nutrition. In Chapter 10, we dig into the significant link that exists between Wand Pilates and nutrition. Within this chapter, we highlight the significance of including a nutritious diet in order to achieve optimal performance, recovery, and general wellness. We discuss nutrition advice that is specifically designed to improve the advantages of Wand Pilates and highlight the significance of maintaining enough water levels in order to support these workouts.

Integrating a Healthy Diet with Wand Pilates:

It is crucial to note that Wand Pilates is not merely a physical exercise; rather, it is a lifestyle that incorporates mindful movement, mental well-being, and, most importantly, a diet that is both balanced and nutritious. When it comes to accomplishing overall health and fitness goals, the synergy that exists between exercise and nutrition is absolutely necessary. The following is an explanation of how individuals can include a healthy diet into their practice of Wand Pilates:

1. **Balanced Macronutrients:**
   - *Protein:* Protein is essential for muscle repair and growth. Incorporate lean protein sources such as poultry, fish, tofu, legumes, and dairy into your diet to support the demands of Wand Pilates. Protein aids in recovery and helps

maintain muscle integrity.

- *Carbohydrates:* Carbohydrates are the body's primary source of energy. Choose complex carbohydrates like whole grains, fruits, and vegetables to provide sustained energy for Pilates sessions. Timing is crucial, and having a balanced mix of macronutrients before and after workouts aids in performance and recovery.

- *Healthy Fats:* Omega-3 fatty acids and other healthy fats contribute to joint health and overall well-being. Include sources like avocados, nuts, seeds, and fatty fish in your diet for improved joint flexibility and cognitive function.

2. **Nutrient-Dense Foods:**

- Prioritize nutrient-dense foods that offer a high concentration of vitamins, minerals, and antioxidants. Colorful fruits and vegetables, whole grains, and lean proteins should form the foundation of your meals to provide the necessary nutrients for energy production and overall health.

3. **Pre-Workout Nutrition:**

- Consume a balanced meal containing carbohydrates, protein, and a moderate amount of healthy fats about 1-2 hours before your Wand Pilates session. This helps fuel your body and ensures sustained energy levels throughout the workout.

4. **Post-Workout Nutrition:**

- After completing a Wand Pilates session, prioritize a post-workout snack or meal rich in protein and carbohydrates. This aids in muscle recovery, replenishes glycogen stores, and supports overall recovery.

5. **Mindful Eating:**

- Apply the principles of mindfulness from Wand Pilates to your eating habits.

Be present and attentive during meals, savoring the flavors and textures of your food. Mindful eating can lead to better digestion and a more intuitive approach to nourishing your body.

Nutrition Tips for Optimal Performance and Recovery:

To enhance the benefits of Wand Pilates and promote optimal performance and recovery, consider the following nutrition tips:

1. **Stay Hydrated:**

   - Proper hydration is fundamental for any physical activity, including Wand Pilates. Water plays a crucial role in maintaining joint lubrication, regulating body temperature, and supporting overall bodily functions. Drink an adequate amount of water throughout the day and consider sipping water during your Pilates session to stay hydrated.

2. **Electrolyte Balance:**

   - Sweating during exercise leads to the loss of electrolytes such as sodium, potassium, and magnesium. Replenish these electrolytes by incorporating foods rich in these minerals into your diet. Additionally, consider electrolyte-rich beverages, especially if you engage in prolonged or intense Wand Pilates sessions.

3. **Incorporate Whole Foods:**

   - Choose whole, minimally processed foods over highly processed options. Whole foods provide a broad spectrum of nutrients that contribute to overall health. Fruits, vegetables, whole grains, lean proteins, and healthy fats should be staples in your diet.

4. **Timing Matters:**

   - Pay attention to the timing of your meals in relation to your Wand Pilates sessions. Eating a balanced meal or snack about 1-2 hours before exercising ensures a readily available energy source. Post-workout nutrition should be consumed within the first hour after exercise to optimize recovery.

5. **Listen to Your Body:**

   - Every individual is unique, and nutritional needs can vary. Pay attention to how your body responds to different foods and adjust your diet accordingly. If you have specific dietary restrictions or health concerns, consult with a healthcare professional or a registered dietitian for personalized guidance.

Hydration and Its Importance in Pilates Workouts:

Hydration is a cornerstone of overall health and plays a crucial role in supporting the demands of Pilates workouts, including Wand Pilates. Here's why staying hydrated is essential for optimal performance and well-being:

1. **Joint Lubrication:**

   - Adequate hydration helps maintain joint lubrication, supporting smooth and fluid movements during Wand Pilates. Proper joint function is vital for executing exercises with precision and reducing the risk of injuries.

2. **Regulating Body Temperature:**

   - Sweating is a natural response to physical activity, including Pilates. Hydration helps regulate body temperature by facilitating the cooling effect of sweating. This is particularly important during more intense or prolonged Wand Pilates sessions.

3. **Energy Production:**

   - Water is involved in numerous metabolic processes, including the production of energy. Staying hydrated ensures that your body can efficiently convert nutrients from food into energy, supporting your performance during Pilates workouts.

4. **Cognitive Function:**

   - Dehydration can negatively impact cognitive function, leading to fatigue and decreased focus. In Wand Pilates, where mindful movement and concentration are key, maintaining optimal cognitive function is essential for getting the most out of each session.

5. **Recovery Support:**

   - Hydration is crucial for the recovery process after exercise. It aids in the transport of nutrients to muscles, helping with muscle repair and glycogen replenishment. Proper hydration contributes to a quicker recovery, allowing you to return to your Wand Pilates practice with renewed energy.

6. **Preventing Fatigue and Cramping:**

   - Dehydration can contribute to muscle fatigue and cramping, which can hinder the effectiveness of your Pilates workout. Ensuring adequate fluid intake helps prevent these issues, promoting a more comfortable and productive exercise experience.

Practical Tips for Staying Hydrated During Wand Pilates:

1. **Pre-Hydration:**

   - Start your day with a glass of water to kickstart hydration. Consider having water before your Wand Pilates session to ensure that you begin in a well-hydrated state.

2. **Carry a Water Bottle:**

   - Keep a reusable water bottle with you throughout the day, making it convenient to sip water regularly. During Wand Pilates, having a water bottle nearby allows for hydration without disrupting the flow of the session.

3. **Hydrate Before You Feel Thirsty:**

   - Thirst is a sign that your body is already in a state of mild dehydration. To stay ahead of this, make a conscious effort to drink water regularly, even if you don't feel thirsty.

4. **Monitor Urine Color:**

   - The color of your urine can provide insights into your hydration status. Aim for pale yellow urine, which indicates adequate hydration. Darker urine may signal dehydration and the need to increase fluid intake.

5. **Include Hydrating Foods:**

   - Certain fruits and vegetables have high water content and can contribute to your overall hydration. Include water-rich foods like watermelon, cucumber, oranges, and celery in your diet.

Chapter 10 has explored the symbiotic relationship between Wand Pilates and nutrition, emphasizing the integration of a healthy diet for optimal performance, recovery, and overall well-being. By paying attention to balanced macronutrients, nutrient-dense foods, and mindful eating, individuals can amplify the benefits of their Wand Pilates practice.

Furthermore, the chapter underscored the importance of hydration in supporting Pilates workouts, highlighting its role in joint lubrication, regulating body temperature, energy production, cognitive function, and recovery. Practical tips for staying hydrated during Wand Pilates sessions were provided to empower individuals to prioritize their hydration needs.

In adopting a holistic approach that combines mindful movement, mental well-being, and a nourishing diet, individuals can unlock the full potential of Wand Pilates, promoting a balanced and vibrant lifestyle. As we conclude this chapter, the message is clear: to truly flourish in Wand Pilates, fuel your body with the nutrients it deserves and hydrate for sustained vitality and optimal performance.

Chapter 11:

Creating Personalized Wand Pilates Routines

The Pilates method is a comprehensive approach to physical training that emphasizes the development of strength, flexibility, and endurance via the use of regulated movements. Because of its adaptability, it is a form of exercise that can be modified to meet the needs of individuals with varied fitness levels and objectives. Within the scope of this chapter, we will investigate the skill of developing individualized wand Pilates routines that are tailored to meet the specific requirements of each individual practitioner.

Designing Individualized Workout Plans:

Understanding the Individual:

After gaining an understanding of the individual's current fitness level, health status, and any particular goals or issues they may have, the first stage in the process of developing a tailored Pilates routine is to collect this information. A comprehensive evaluation should take into account a variety of aspects, including flexibility, strength, balance, and any injuries or limits that may already be present. The foundation upon which a customized exercise routine might be constructed is contained within this material.

Tailoring Exercises to Specific Goals:

A vast variety of exercises that target different muscle groups and fitness components are included in the Pilates workout program. It is possible to tailor the routine to place an emphasis on particular exercises, depending on the objectives of the individual, which may include improving core strength, flexibility, rehabilitation, or general fitness goals. As an illustration, an individual who is interested in enhancing their core strength would concentrate on exercises such as the Hundred, variations of the Plank, and the Saw.

Considering Physical Limitations:

In the process of developing a personalized Pilates practice, it is essential to take into consideration any physical restrictions or health concerns that may exist. In order to accommodate persons who have injuries or diseases such as osteoporosis or arthritis, exercises can be modified or substituted using alternative methods. A competent Pilates instructor should be familiar with the process of modifying routines in order to guarantee that everyone receives a workout that is both safe and effective.

Incorporating Variety:

In order to maintain the routine's effectiveness and interest, it is essential to incorporate a range of methods. In addition to preventing boredom, this guarantees that different muscle groups are continually engaged, which is a significant benefit. A new dimension can be added to the workout by incorporating props such as the Pilates wand. These props provide resistance and target specific muscle areas in a manner that is very different from other methods.

Gradual Progression:

When developing a personalized Pilates regimen, it is important to take into account the individual's present level of fitness and to progressively increase the intensity of the movements. It is important that the routine evolves to meet the practitioner's developing strength and endurance. This can be accomplished by increasing the number of repetitions, the resistance, or the incorporation of more challenging variations.

Setting Realistic Goals and Tracking Progress:

Establishing Clear Objectives:

When it comes to keeping oneself motivated and keeping track of one's progress, setting goals that are both reasonable and attainable is vital. These objectives may be short-term, such as becoming proficient in a particular Pilates motion, or they may be long-term, such as progressing toward an overall improvement in fitness. The individual is provided with a road map in the form of clearly defined objectives, which also serve as milestones which can be celebrated along the fitness journey.

Monitoring and Adjusting Goals:

Regular assessment and feedback sessions are crucial to track progress and adjust goals accordingly. As the individual advances in their Pilates practice, goals may need to be modified to align with their evolving capabilities and aspirations. This adaptive approach ensures that the routine remains challenging and effective.

Utilizing Technology:

In the digital age, technology can play a significant role in goal tracking. Fitness apps, wearables, and online platforms can help individuals monitor their workouts, track progress, and receive feedback. Integrating these tools into the personalized Pilates routine enhances the overall experience and provides valuable insights into performance metrics.

Celebrating Achievements:

Acknowledging and celebrating achievements, no matter how small, is vital for maintaining motivation. Whether it's mastering a challenging exercise or reaching a specific fitness milestone, recognizing and celebrating these accomplishments reinforces the individual's commitment to their Pilates practice.

Adapting Routines to Changing Fitness Levels:

Dynamic Assessment:

Fitness is dynamic, and an individual's capabilities can change over time. Regular reassessment of fitness levels allows for adjustments to the Pilates routine. This can involve modifying exercises, introducing new challenges, or addressing any emerging concerns or limitations.

Aging Gracefully:

As individuals age, their fitness needs and abilities evolve. A personalized Pilates routine can be adapted to address the changing requirements of aging bodies. Emphasizing flexibility, balance, and joint mobility becomes increasingly important, and the routine can be tailored to promote overall well-being.

Post-Injury Rehabilitation:

For those recovering from injuries, Pilates can be a valuable tool for rehabilitation. The routine can be customized to focus on strengthening specific areas, improving flexibility, and promoting a gradual return to full functionality. A collaborative approach with healthcare professionals ensures a safe and effective recovery process.

Cross-Training Integration:

To prevent plateaus and promote overall fitness, integrating cross-training elements into the Pilates routine can be beneficial. This may involve incorporating cardiovascular exercises, resistance training, or other forms of movement that complement the Pilates practice. The personalized routine becomes a holistic approach to fitness that addresses multiple dimensions of well-being.

Mind-Body Connection:

Adapting Pilates routines goes beyond the physical aspects; it also involves nurturing the mind-body connection. Incorporating mindfulness and relaxation techniques into the routine can help manage stress, improve mental focus, and enhance the overall experience of Pilates. This holistic approach contributes to a well-rounded and sustainable fitness practice.

Creating personalized wand Pilates routines requires a thoughtful and individualized approach. By understanding the unique needs, goals, and limitations of each practitioner, instructors can design routines that are not only effective but also enjoyable. Setting realistic goals, tracking progress, and adapting to changing fitness levels are essential components of a successful and sustainable Pilates practice. As the personalized routine evolves with the individual, it becomes a dynamic tool for promoting overall health, fitness, and well-being.

Chapter 12:

Wand Pilates in a Group Setting:

Throughout the years, Pilates has developed to integrate a wide variety of props and pieces of equipment. Pilates is a kind of exercise that focuses on strength, flexibility, and general body awareness. The wand is one example of a prop that has become increasingly popular in some Pilates courses. These Pilates exercises are made more difficult and effective by the addition of the wand, which is a tool that is both simple and versatile. It adds a layer of resistance and control to the exercises. In this chapter, we will discuss the mechanics of leading group Pilates sessions with wands, with a particular emphasis on the significance of community, support, and the ability to alter exercises for persons who have varying degrees of fitness.

Leading Group Classes with Wands:

Engaging participants in a group environment through the use of Wand Pilates sessions is an interesting and new approach to motivate them. To add an additional element of difficulty, the usage of wands necessitates that players concentrate on maintaining control, maintaining stability, and maintaining precision. As an instructor, it is of the utmost importance to design a class that is well-structured and that meets the varied requirements of the participants while also preserving a sense of cooperation among the members of the group.

1. **Class Structure and Planning:** A well-planned and organized class framework is very necessary in order to successfully include wands into a group Pilates session.

Let's start off with a little warm-up to get the body ready for the workouts that are about to come. Exercises such as dynamic stretches, breathing exercises, and modest joint mobilization could be included in this category. The majority of the lesson should be comprised of a series of exercises that are particular to the use of wands and target various muscle groups and movement patterns of the participants. At long last, bring the session to a close with a cool-down portion that emphasizes flexibility and relaxation respectively.

2. **Sequencing and Progressions:** In a Wand Pilates class, the order in which exercises are performed is quite important. Beginning with foundational movements that allow participants to become familiar with the wand and its role in enhancing their Pilates experience is a good place to start. Participants should be gradually introduced to more difficult activities that test their strength, coordination, and balance as the session develops. It is important to provide changes and progressions to accommodate different levels of fitness, so that everyone can feel like they are being appropriately pushed.

3. **Cueing and Alignment:** When teaching a Wand Pilates class, it is essential to provide cues that are both clear and accurate. In order to comprehend the movement patterns and ensure that they are maintained in the correct alignment, the participants rely on your spoken directions. Throughout the entirety of the session, stress the significance of maintaining core engagement, practicing correct breathing methods, and being aware of your body. In order to maintain a good and welcoming atmosphere, you should adjust your cues in accordance with the feedback and replies provided by the participants.

Encouraging Community and Support:

Developing a sense of community among the participants in a Pilates class is absolutely necessary in order to cultivate an environment that is upbeat and encouraging. When participants work together toward a common objective of improved strength, flexibility, and overall well-being, the usage of wands can enhance this communal experience and make it more enjoyable for everyone involved.

1. **Group Dynamics:** Activities that include the usage of wands should be incorporated into pair or small group activities. Not only does this provide a fun element to the event, but it also encourages attendees to get together and form connections with one another. The dynamics of the group can help to cultivate a sense of camaraderie, which in turn can make the session more fun and motivating for all of the individuals engaged.

2. **Shared Goals and Achievements:** Set goals that everyone in the class can agree on, and then celebrate everyone's successes together. The mastery of a difficult wand exercise, the improvement of flexibility, or the accomplishment of a personal fitness milestone are all excellent examples of this. Creating a supportive environment in which participants feel appreciated and driven can be accomplished by recognizing the work of individuals within the context of the group setting.

3. **Open Communication:** It is important to encourage open communication among both parties. Make it possible for people to talk about their experiences, the difficulties they faced, and the victories they achieved. This may be accomplished through brief discussions at the beginning or end of the class, or by introducing a

brief social time during which participants have the opportunity to engage with one another and create relationships that extend beyond the workout.

Modifying Exercises for Various Fitness Levels:

Individuals that participate in a group environment bring with them a wide range of fitness levels, abilities, and existing experiences. As a Pilates instructor, it is your duty to offer modifications and alternatives to ensure that every participant is able to participate in the class in a manner that is both successful and respectful of their specific requirements and constraints.

1. Individualized Attention and Assessment: To begin, it is important to evaluate the participants' current levels of physical fitness and any potential limits they may have. It is important to provide individualized attention, particularly to individuals who may be new to the process or who have particular concerns. As you move around the classroom, observe the participants' performances and provide them with individualized feedback to improve their overall experience.

2. Progressions and Alterations to the System: Wand The movements in Pilates can be easily modified or progressed to accommodate individuals with varying degrees of fitness readiness. There should be simplified versions of workouts that have less resistance or range of motion for those who are just starting out. Once the participants have reached a point where they are more comfortable, progressively introduce progressions that are more difficult for them. Because of this, it is guaranteed that every single person in the class, regardless of their previous fitness level, will be suitably pushed.

3. Terminology that is Inclusive: Make use of language that is inclusive and

acknowledges the variety of fitness levels that are present within the group. Make sure to remind the participants that it is completely fine to adapt the exercises in accordance with their level of comfort and competence. This results in the creation of a non-judgmental atmosphere in which individuals feel empowered to make decisions that are tailored to their specific requirements.

Wand Pilates, when performed in a group setting, offers an exercise experience that is not only dynamic and engaging but also unique in comparison to regular mat Pilates. Not only is it your responsibility as an instructor to lead participants through the exercises, but you are also responsible for fostering a sense of community, support, and inclusivity within the environment of the class. Through the implementation of well-planned lessons, the promotion of open communication, and the provision of adaptations, you are able to establish a setting in which individuals of varying fitness levels are able to flourish and reap the multiple advantages that Wand Pilates has to offer.

Conclusion

During the enthralling voyage that we took through the pages of "Wand Pilates," we went on an in-depth investigation of many aspects of the mind, body, and soul. A comprehensive approach to health and wellness has been made possible as a result of this one-of-a-kind combination of old knowledge and contemporary comprehension. As we come to the end of our literary journey, let us take a moment to revive the spirit of our journey and embody the essence of Wand Pilates.

This book has been a zealous champion for the harmonious synchronization of the mind and body, using the wand as a conduit to connect with the deep reservoirs of our inner strength. At its core, this book has been a fierce supporter for this. This is not only a set of exercises; rather, it is a way of life that goes beyond the surface limitations of fitness. The practice of Wand Pilates is a tribute to the fundamental link that exists between our physical and mental well-being. It is a dance between the tangible and the intangible, a symphony of movement and mindfulness.

Throughout the course of our journey, we delved into the profound philosophy that underpins Wand Pilates, peeling back the layers of its beginnings and passing down the knowledge that has been passed down from generation to generation. The creation of a discipline that extends beyond the bounds of traditional exercise was something that we witnessed. From the distant echoes of ancient practices to the present incorporation of Pilates principles, we witnessed the evolution of this discipline. This event is a celebration of resiliency and a monument to the everlasting spirit of adaptability that is inside humans.

As we made our way through the maze of our investigation, we made our way through the intricate tapestry of Pilates positions, with each movement serving as a stroke of the brush on the canvas of self-discovery. Each each chapter revealed a new facet of our potential, beginning with the fundamental exercises that establish a foundation for strength and stability and progressing to the more complex sequences that test our limitations. We realized that the wand was more than simply a piece of equipment; it was also a buddy that helped us navigate the rhythmic flow of breath and action.

The pledge that was made at the outset of this journey was not only a commitment to health and fitness in the physical realm; rather, it was a covenant to overall well-being. It is becoming increasingly clear that the solution that is being presented here goes beyond the limitations of an exercise routine as we reflect on the pages that have been turned and the postures that have been assumed. The practice of Wand Pilates extends an invitation to adopt a way of life that fosters the mutually beneficial interaction that exists between our physical vigor and mental equilibrium.

There were obstacles along the way that we had to overcome. We overcame the challenges of self-doubt and physical limits, and as a result, we emerged from the experience more powerful and more attuned to the utterances of our inner selves. The wand, when used with elegance and intention, transformed into an instrument for empowerment, a catalyst for the transformation that takes place when we match our actions with our aspirations.

In light of the fact that we are rapidly approaching the end of this discussion, it is of the utmost importance to condense the essence of Wand Pilates into a single takeaway. Among the rich trove of these pages, if there is one jewel that you should take with you, let it be the knowledge that genuine well-being extends beyond the physical realm. It refers to the harmonious combination of the mind, the body, and the spirit. Wand Pilates is not simply a practice; it is a philosophy, a way of life that encourages you to step into your authenticity, embrace your strength, and relish in the flow of your being. Wand Pilates is a way of life.

The practice of Wand Pilates emerges as a silent guide, a whisper that begs us to return to ourselves, in the immense fabric of existence, where confusion and tumult frequently obscure the voice that resides inside. We discover a sanctuary where the clamor of the outside world melts away, and we are left with the purity of our essence. This sanctuary is found through the undulating motions and the constant rhythm of the breath.

It is my hope that the reverberations of Wand Pilates will continue to reverberate in the hallways of your awareness when we part ways with this literary companion. I wish for the lessons that you take away from your time spent on the mat to seep into the fabric of your everyday life, imbuing each moment with intention and present. Allow this to be more than just a conclusion; allow it to be an invitation to a journey of self-discovery that will last a lifetime, one in which the wand becomes not only an instrument of movement but also a wand of transformation, directing you toward the most complete expression of your radiant self.